MULTIPLE MYELOMA CANCER
COOKBOOK

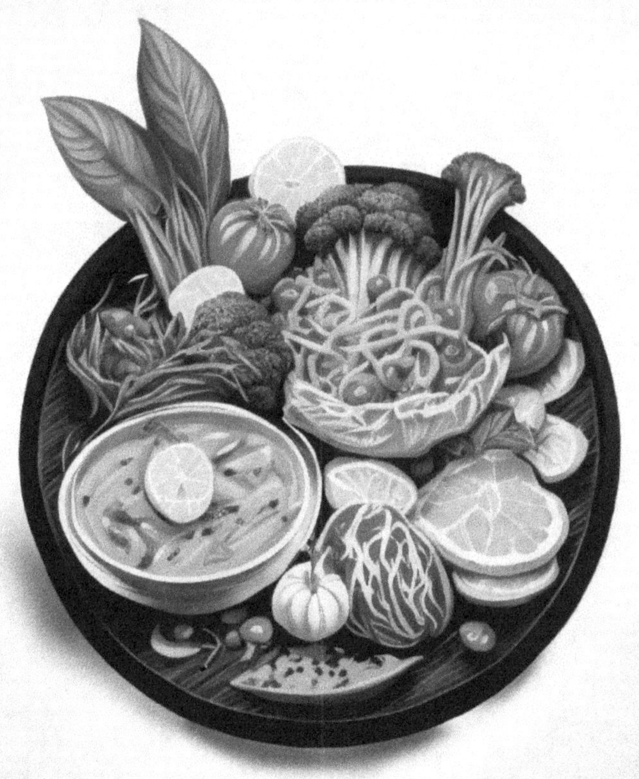

GET READY, LET'S FIGHT!

THIS BOOK BELONGS TO

Multiple Myeloma Cancer Cookbook

==============================

Feeding Hope, Nurturing Health

Jetta Harlow Olson

Attribution: The resources utilized to design this cover were obtained from pexels.com.

ISBN: 9798857970331

Imprint: Independently Published

Disclaimer

This book's instructions, recommendations, or methods are not intended to replace professional medical guidance, diagnosis, or care. The information in this book is only meant to be used for educational purposes; it should not be used as a replacement for professional medical advice from a healthcare provider.

The authors and publisher of this book disclaim any responsibility for any negative effects or outcomes attributable to the use of the knowledge, suggestions, or methods offered in this book. Readers should speak with their doctor before beginning any new health or wellness program.

Despite the fact that the knowledge and research upon which the information in this book is based is up-to-date, medical procedures and recommendations may alter over time.

It is advised that readers seek out additional information and keep current with healthcare trends.

The authors' views are the only ones that are expressed in this book; they do not necessarily represent the publisher's views. The authors and publisher do not endorse or recommend any companies, items, or services that are mentioned in this book.

Despite making every effort to ensure the accuracy and comprehensiveness of the information in this book, the authors and publisher make no promises or representations of any kind, either explicitly or implicitly, regarding the information's suitability, reliability, or availability.

Any risks associated with relying on the information in this book are assumed by the reader.

Contents

1. Personal Motivation for the Cookbook

Creating a cookbook focused on nutritious and delicious recipes for individuals with multiple myeloma holds a deeply personal significance for me. As someone who has witnessed the challenges that cancer patients and their loved ones face, I am driven by the desire to offer practical support during their journey.

My own experience with cancer has fostered a strong sense of empathy and understanding. I have seen firsthand the impact that a well-balanced diet can have on managing symptoms, boosting energy levels, and enhancing overall well-being. By compiling a collection of recipes tailored to the unique dietary needs of multiple myeloma patients, I hope to provide a source of comfort, empowerment, and inspiration.

The cookbook is not just about recipes; it's a beacon of hope and a reminder that nourishing the body is an essential part of the healing process. I am motivated to contribute positively to the lives of those affected by multiple myeloma, to offer caregivers practical tools to provide comfort through food, and to create a sense of community and solidarity through shared experiences.

Seeing individuals embrace these recipes and find joy in preparing and enjoying them fuels my motivation. Each recipe is carefully crafted to offer a blend of flavors, nutrients, and textures that cater to various dietary requirements, ensuring that individuals with multiple myeloma can enjoy their meals while receiving the essential nutrients their bodies need.

In this cookbook, I strive to share my passion for cooking, my understanding of the challenges cancer patients face, and my commitment to supporting their well-being. By bringing these elements together, I hope to make a meaningful contribution to the lives of those touched by multiple myeloma, helping them navigate their journey with strength, nourishment, and a renewed sense of hope.

Important Note: These recipes offer a variety of nutrient-rich ingredients and cater to different dietary preferences. Remember to tailor the portion sizes and ingredients to suit individual needs and dietary restrictions. Always consult with a healthcare professional before making significant changes to a patient's diet, especially for individuals undergoing cancer treatment.

2. Creamy Quinoa Breakfast Bowl

Ingredients:

- 1/2 cup quinoa, rinsed
- 1 cup almond milk
- 1 ripe banana, mashed
- 1 tablespoon chia seeds
- 1/4 teaspoon cinnamon
- Toppings: mixed berries, chopped nuts, honey

Instructions:

1. In a small saucepan, combine quinoa and almond milk. Bring to a boil, then reduce heat and simmer for 15-20 minutes, or until quinoa is cooked and liquid is absorbed.

2. Stir in mashed banana, chia seeds, and cinnamon.

3. Serve in bowls, topped with mixed berries, chopped nuts, and a drizzle of honey.

3. Roasted Vegetable and Lentil Salad

Ingredients:

- 1 cup green or brown lentils, cooked and drained

- Assorted vegetables (e.g., bell peppers, zucchini, cherry tomatoes), chopped

- 2 tablespoons olive oil

- 1 teaspoon dried herbs (thyme, oregano, rosemary)

- Salt and pepper to taste

- Lemon vinaigrette: lemon juice, olive oil, Dijon mustard

Instructions:

1. Preheat oven to 400°F (200°C).

2. Toss chopped vegetables with olive oil, dried herbs, salt, and pepper. Roast in the oven until tender and slightly caramelized.

3. In a large bowl, combine cooked lentils and roasted vegetables.

4. Drizzle with lemon vinaigrette and toss gently before serving.

4. Ginger-Turmeric Carrot Soup

Ingredients:

- 1 pound carrots, peeled and chopped
- 1 onion, chopped
- 2 cloves garlic, minced
- 1-inch piece of ginger, peeled and grated
- 1 teaspoon ground turmeric
- 4 cups vegetable broth
- 1 cup coconut milk
- Salt and pepper to taste
- Fresh cilantro for garnish

Instructions:

1. In a large pot, sauté chopped onion, garlic, and ginger until fragrant.
2. Add chopped carrots, ground turmeric, and vegetable broth. Bring to a boil, then reduce heat and simmer until carrots are tender.
3. Use an immersion blender to puree the soup until smooth.
4. Stir in coconut milk and season with salt and pepper. Heat gently without boiling.

5. Serve hot, garnished with fresh cilantro.

5. Baked Salmon with Herbed Quinoa

Ingredients:

- 2 salmon fillets

- 1 tablespoon olive oil

- Lemon zest and juice

- Salt and pepper to taste

- 1 cup quinoa, rinsed

- Fresh herbs (such as parsley, dill, chives), chopped

Instructions:

1. Preheat oven to 375°F (190°C).

2. Place salmon fillets on a baking sheet. Drizzle with olive oil and lemon juice, then sprinkle with lemon zest, salt, and pepper.

3. Bake for about 15-20 minutes, or until salmon flakes easily with a fork.

4. While the salmon is baking, cook quinoa according to package instructions. Stir in fresh herbs.

5. Serve salmon over a bed of herbed quinoa.

6. Spinach and Berry Salad with Citrus Vinaigrette

Ingredients:

- 4 cups baby spinach

- 1 cup mixed berries (strawberries, blueberries, raspberries)

- 1/4 cup chopped walnuts

- Crumbled feta cheese (optional)

For Citrus Vinaigrette:

- 2 tablespoons olive oil

- 2 tablespoons fresh orange juice

- 1 tablespoon fresh lemon juice

- 1 teaspoon honey

- Salt and pepper to taste

Instructions:

1. In a large bowl, combine baby spinach, mixed berries, and chopped walnuts.

2. In a small bowl, whisk together the olive oil, orange juice, lemon juice, honey, salt, and pepper.

3. Drizzle the vinaigrette over the salad and toss gently to combine.

4. If desired, sprinkle crumbled feta cheese on top before serving.

7. Lemon Herb Grilled Chicken

Ingredients:

- 2 boneless, skinless chicken breasts

- 2 tablespoons olive oil

- Zest and juice of 1 lemon

- 2 cloves garlic, minced

- 1 teaspoon dried thyme

- Salt and pepper to taste

Instructions:

1. In a bowl, whisk together olive oil, lemon zest, lemon juice, minced garlic, dried thyme, salt, and pepper.

2. Place the chicken breasts in a resealable plastic bag and pour the marinade over them. Seal the bag and refrigerate for at least 30 minutes.

3. Preheat a grill or grill pan over medium-high heat. Grill the chicken for about 6-7 minutes per side, or until cooked through.

4. Let the chicken rest for a few minutes before slicing. Serve with your choice of sides.

8. Butternut Squash and Red Lentil Stew

Ingredients:

- 2 cups butternut squash, peeled and cubed
- 1 cup red lentils, rinsed
- 1 onion, chopped
- 2 cloves garlic, minced
- 1 teaspoon ground cumin
- 1/2 teaspoon ground coriander
- 4 cups vegetable broth
- 1 cup coconut milk
- Fresh cilantro for garnish

Instructions:

1. In a large pot, sauté chopped onion and minced garlic until softened.

2. Add cubed butternut squash, red lentils, ground cumin, and ground coriander. Stir to combine.

3. Pour in vegetable broth and bring to a boil. Reduce heat and simmer until the squash and lentils are tender.

4. Use an immersion blender to partially puree the stew, leaving some texture.

5. Stir in coconut milk and heat gently. Season with salt and pepper.

6. Serve the stew hot, garnished with fresh cilantro.

9. Oatmeal Banana Muffins

Ingredients:

- 2 ripe bananas, mashed

- 2 eggs

- 1/4 cup honey or maple syrup

- 1/4 cup Greek yogurt

- 1 teaspoon vanilla extract

- 1 1/2 cups oats

- 1 teaspoon baking powder

- 1/2 teaspoon cinnamon

- 1/4 teaspoon salt

- Optional mix-ins: chopped nuts, raisins, dark chocolate chips

Instructions:

1. Preheat the oven to 350°F (175°C) and line a muffin tin with paper liners.

2. In a bowl, whisk together mashed bananas, eggs, honey or maple syrup, Greek yogurt, and vanilla extract.

3. In another bowl, combine oats, baking powder, cinnamon, and salt.

4. Mix the wet and dry ingredients until well combined. If using, fold in the optional mix-ins.

5. Divide the batter evenly among the muffin cups.

6. Bake for about 20-25 minutes, or until a toothpick inserted into the center comes out clean.

7. Allow the muffins to cool in the tin for a few minutes before transferring to a wire rack to cool completely.

10.Quinoa and Roasted Vegetable Stuffed Bell Peppers

Ingredients:

- 4 bell peppers, tops removed and seeds removed

- 1 cup cooked quinoa

- Assorted roasted vegetables (such as bell peppers, zucchini, eggplant)

- 1/2 cup crumbled feta cheese

- Fresh basil or parsley for garnish

Instructions:

1. Preheat the oven to 375°F (190°C).

2. In a bowl, combine cooked quinoa, roasted vegetables, and crumbled feta cheese.

3. Stuff each bell pepper with the quinoa and vegetable mixture.

4. Place the stuffed peppers in a baking dish and bake for about 20-25 minutes, or until the peppers are tender.

5. Garnish with fresh basil or parsley before serving.

11.Creamy Avocado and White Bean Dip

Ingredients:

- 1 can (15 oz) white beans, drained and rinsed

- 1 ripe avocado, peeled and pitted

- 2 cloves garlic, minced

- Juice of 1 lemon

- 2 tablespoons olive oil

- Salt and pepper to taste

- Optional toppings: red pepper flakes, chopped fresh herbs

Instructions:

1. In a food processor, combine white beans, avocado, minced garlic, lemon juice, and olive oil.

2. Blend until smooth and creamy. If needed, add a splash of water to achieve desired consistency.

3. Season with salt and pepper to taste.

4. Transfer the dip to a serving bowl and top with red pepper flakes and chopped fresh herbs, if desired.

5. Serve with sliced vegetables or whole grain crackers.

12.Baked Sweet Potato Fries

Ingredients:

- 2 large sweet potatoes, peeled and cut into fries

- 2 tablespoons olive oil

- 1 teaspoon paprika

- 1/2 teaspoon garlic powder

- Salt and pepper to taste

Instructions:

1. Preheat the oven to 425°F (220°C) and line a baking sheet with parchment paper.

2. In a bowl, toss sweet potato fries with olive oil, paprika, garlic powder, salt, and pepper until evenly coated.

3. Spread the fries in a single layer on the prepared baking sheet.

4. Bake for about 20-25 minutes, flipping halfway through, until the fries are crispy and golden brown.

5. Serve the sweet potato fries as a side dish or snack.

13.Chia Seed Pudding with Berries

Ingredients:

- 1/4 cup chia seeds
- 1 cup almond milk (or any milk of choice)
- 1 tablespoon honey or maple syrup
- 1/2 teaspoon vanilla extract
- Mixed berries for topping

Instructions:

1. In a jar or bowl, whisk together chia seeds, almond milk, honey or maple syrup, and vanilla extract.

2. Cover and refrigerate for at least 4 hours or overnight, allowing the mixture to thicken.

3. Before serving, give the chia pudding a good stir to break up any clumps.

4. Serve the chia seed pudding in bowls, topped with mixed berries.

14. Grilled Vegetable Quinoa Salad

Ingredients:

- 1 cup quinoa, rinsed

- Assorted grilled vegetables (such as bell peppers, eggplant, asparagus)

- 1/4 cup chopped fresh herbs (parsley, mint, basil)

- 1/4 cup crumbled goat cheese (optional)

- Lemon vinaigrette: lemon juice, olive oil, Dijon mustard, honey

Instructions:

1. Cook quinoa according to package instructions and let it cool.

2. Combine cooked quinoa with grilled vegetables and chopped fresh herbs in a large bowl.

3. Drizzle with lemon vinaigrette and toss gently to combine.

4. If desired, sprinkle crumbled goat cheese on top before serving.

15.Turmeric Ginger Smoothie

Ingredients:

- 1 cup unsweetened almond milk (or any milk of choice)
- 1 ripe banana
- 1/2 cup frozen mango chunks
- 1 teaspoon turmeric powder
- 1/2 teaspoon grated fresh ginger
- 1 tablespoon chia seeds or flaxseeds
- Optional: honey or maple syrup to sweeten

Instructions:

1. Combine almond milk, banana, frozen mango, turmeric, ginger, and chia seeds in a blender.
2. Blend until smooth and creamy.
3. Taste and add honey or maple syrup if desired.
4. Pour the smoothie into a glass and enjoy.

16.Roasted Chicken and Vegetable Quinoa Bowl

Ingredients:

- 2 boneless, skinless chicken breasts

- Assorted vegetables (such as broccoli, carrots, bell peppers)

- 1 cup cooked quinoa

- Olive oil

- Garlic powder, onion powder, dried oregano

- Salt and pepper to taste

Instructions:

1. Preheat the oven to 400°F (200°C).

2. Season chicken breasts with garlic powder, onion powder, dried oregano, salt, and pepper.

3. Toss chopped vegetables with olive oil, salt, and pepper.

4. Place chicken breasts and vegetables on a baking sheet. Bake for about 20-25 minutes, or until chicken is cooked through and vegetables are roasted.

5. Slice the chicken and serve it over cooked quinoa with roasted vegetables.

17.Berry Chia Jam

Ingredients:

- 2 cups mixed berries (strawberries, blueberries, raspberries)

- 2 tablespoons chia seeds

- 1-2 tablespoons honey or maple syrup (adjust to taste)

- Juice of 1 lemon

Instructions:

1. In a saucepan, heat mixed berries over medium heat until they start to break down and release juices.

2. Mash the berries with a fork or potato masher to desired consistency.

3. Stir in chia seeds, honey or maple syrup, and lemon juice.

4. Continue to cook for a few more minutes until the mixture thickens.

5. Remove from heat and let the jam cool. Transfer to a jar and refrigerate.

18. Mediterranean Chickpea Salad

Ingredients:

- 2 cups cooked chickpeas (canned or cooked from dried)

- 1 cup cherry tomatoes, halved

- 1 cucumber, diced

- 1/4 red onion, thinly sliced

- Kalamata olives, pitted and sliced

- Crumbled feta cheese (optional)

- Fresh parsley, chopped

For Lemon Herb Dressing:

- 3 tablespoons olive oil

- Juice of 1 lemon

- 1 teaspoon dried oregano

- Salt and pepper to taste

Instructions:

1. In a large bowl, combine chickpeas, cherry tomatoes, cucumber, red onion, olives, and feta cheese.

2. In a small bowl, whisk together olive oil, lemon juice, dried oregano, salt, and pepper.

3. Drizzle the dressing over the salad and toss gently.

4. Garnish with fresh parsley before serving.

19. Baked Cod with Herbed Quinoa and Asparagus

Ingredients:

- 2 cod fillets

- 2 tablespoons olive oil

- Lemon zest and juice

- Salt and pepper to taste

- 1 cup quinoa, cooked

- Fresh herbs (such as dill, parsley), chopped

- Asparagus spears, trimmed

Instructions:

1. Preheat the oven to 375°F (190°C).

2. Place cod fillets on a baking sheet. Drizzle with olive oil and lemon juice, then sprinkle with lemon zest, salt, and pepper.

3. Arrange asparagus spears around the cod on the baking sheet.

4. Bake for about 12-15 minutes, or until the cod flakes easily with a fork.

5. While the fish is baking, mix chopped fresh herbs into the cooked quinoa.

6. Serve the baked cod over a bed of herbed quinoa with roasted asparagus.

20. Creamy Broccoli Soup

Ingredients:

- 2 cups broccoli florets

- 1 onion, chopped

- 2 cloves garlic, minced

- 1 potato, peeled and diced

- 4 cups vegetable broth

- 1/2 cup unsweetened almond milk (or any milk of choice)

- Salt and pepper to taste

Instructions:

1. In a large pot, sauté chopped onion and minced garlic until translucent.

2. Add diced potato, broccoli florets, and vegetable broth. Bring to a boil, then reduce heat and simmer until vegetables are tender.

3. Use an immersion blender to puree the soup until smooth.

4. Stir in almond milk and heat gently. Season with salt and pepper.

5. Serve the creamy broccoli soup hot.

21.Apple Cinnamon Oat Bars

Ingredients:

- 2 cups old-fashioned oats

- 1 cup applesauce

- 1/4 cup almond butter (or any nut/seed butter)

- 1/4 cup honey or maple syrup

- 1 teaspoon ground cinnamon

- 1/2 cup dried fruits (raisins, chopped dates) and/or chopped nuts

Instructions:

1. Preheat the oven to 350°F (175°C) and line a baking dish with parchment paper.

2. In a bowl, combine oats, applesauce, almond butter, honey or maple syrup, and ground cinnamon.

3. Mix in dried fruits and/or nuts.

4. Press the mixture evenly into the prepared baking dish.

5. Bake for about 25-30 minutes, or until the bars are golden and set.

6. Let the bars cool before cutting into squares.

22.Lentil and Vegetable Stir-Fry

Ingredients:

- 1 cup green or brown lentils, cooked

- Assorted stir-fry vegetables (bell peppers, broccoli, carrots, snap peas)

- 2 tablespoons low-sodium soy sauce or tamari

- 1 tablespoon sesame oil

- 1 teaspoon grated fresh ginger

- 2 cloves garlic, minced

- Optional: chopped cashews or almonds for garnish

Instructions:

1. In a wok or large skillet, heat sesame oil over medium-high heat.

2. Add grated ginger and minced garlic, and sauté briefly until fragrant.

3. Add the stir-fry vegetables and cook until they begin to soften.

4. Stir in cooked lentils and continue to cook for a few more minutes.

5. Drizzle soy sauce or tamari over the mixture and toss to combine.

6. Serve the lentil and vegetable stir-fry with optional chopped nuts on top.

23.Berry and Spinach Smoothie Bowl

Ingredients:

- 1 cup fresh spinach leaves

- 1/2 cup mixed berries (strawberries, blueberries, raspberries)

- 1/2 banana

- 1/2 cup unsweetened almond milk (or any milk of choice)

- Toppings: sliced banana, granola, chia seeds, shredded coconut

Instructions:

1. Blend spinach, mixed berries, banana, and almond milk until smooth.

2. Pour the smoothie into a bowl.

3. Top with sliced banana, granola, chia seeds, and shredded coconut for added texture and nutrients.

4. Enjoy the smoothie bowl with a spoon.

24.Roasted Cauliflower and Chickpea Tacos

Ingredients:

- 2 cups cauliflower florets

- 1 can (15 oz) chickpeas, drained and rinsed

- 1 tablespoon olive oil

- 1 teaspoon ground cumin

- 1/2 teaspoon smoked paprika

- Salt and pepper to taste

- Whole grain tortillas

- Toppings: avocado slices, salsa, Greek yogurt, cilantro

Instructions:

1. Preheat the oven to 400°F (200°C).

2. Toss cauliflower florets and chickpeas with olive oil, ground cumin, smoked paprika, salt, and pepper.

3. Spread the mixture on a baking sheet and roast for about 20-25 minutes, or until the cauliflower is tender and slightly crispy.

4. Warm the tortillas.

5. Assemble the tacos with the roasted cauliflower and chickpeas, and top with avocado slices, salsa, Greek yogurt, and cilantro.

25. Coconut Rice Pudding with Mango

Ingredients:

- 1 cup cooked white rice

- 1 can (13.5 oz) coconut milk

- 2 tablespoons honey or maple syrup

- 1 teaspoon vanilla extract

- Pinch of salt

- Fresh mango slices for topping

- Optional: toasted coconut flakes

Instructions:

1. In a saucepan, combine cooked rice, coconut milk, honey or maple syrup, vanilla extract, and a pinch of salt.

2. Cook over medium heat, stirring occasionally, until the mixture thickens and becomes creamy.

3. Remove from heat and let the rice pudding cool slightly.

4. Serve in bowls, topped with fresh mango slices and toasted coconut flakes if desired.

26.Quinoa-Stuffed Bell Peppers

Ingredients:

- 4 large bell peppers, tops removed and seeds removed

- 1 cup cooked quinoa

- 1 can (15 oz) black beans, drained and rinsed

- 1 cup corn kernels (fresh, frozen, or canned)

- 1 cup diced tomatoes (canned or fresh)

- 1 teaspoon cumin

- 1/2 teaspoon chili powder

- Salt and pepper to taste

- Grated cheese (cheddar or vegan alternative), for topping

Instructions:

1. Preheat the oven to 375°F (190°C).

2. In a bowl, combine cooked quinoa, black beans, corn, diced tomatoes, cumin, chili powder, salt, and pepper.

3. Stuff each bell pepper with the quinoa mixture.

4. Place the stuffed peppers in a baking dish. Top with grated cheese.

5. Cover with aluminum foil and bake for about 25-30 minutes. Remove the foil and bake for an additional 10 minutes, until the cheese is melted and bubbly.

6. Allow the stuffed peppers to cool slightly before serving.

27. Cucumber and Dill Greek Yogurt Dip

Ingredients:

- 1 cup Greek yogurt

- 1 cucumber, finely grated and drained

- 2 tablespoons fresh dill, chopped

- 1 clove garlic, minced

- Juice of 1 lemon

- Salt and pepper to taste

Instructions:

1. In a bowl, combine Greek yogurt, grated cucumber, chopped dill, minced garlic, and lemon juice.

2. Mix well and season with salt and pepper to taste.

3. Refrigerate the dip for at least 30 minutes before serving.

4. Serve with vegetable sticks, whole grain crackers, or pita bread.

28.Mushroom and Spinach Frittata

Ingredients:

- 6 large eggs
- 1 cup sliced mushrooms
- 2 cups fresh spinach leaves
- 1/2 onion, chopped
- 1/4 cup grated Parmesan cheese (optional)
- Salt and pepper to taste
- Olive oil for cooking

Instructions:

1. Preheat the oven to 350°F (175°C).

2. In a skillet, sauté chopped onion and sliced mushrooms in olive oil until softened.

3. Add fresh spinach and cook until wilted.

4. In a bowl, whisk eggs, grated Parmesan cheese, salt, and pepper.

5. Pour the egg mixture into the skillet over the vegetables.

6. Cook on the stovetop for a few minutes until the edges set.

7. Transfer the skillet to the preheated oven and bake for about 15-20 minutes, until the frittata is cooked through and slightly puffed.

8. Let the frittata cool slightly before slicing and serving.

29.Banana Nut Oat Muffins

Ingredients:

- 2 ripe bananas, mashed

- 1/4 cup coconut oil, melted

- 1/4 cup honey or maple syrup

- 2 eggs

- 1 teaspoon vanilla extract

- 1 1/2 cups oats

- 1 teaspoon baking powder

- 1/2 teaspoon cinnamon

- 1/4 teaspoon salt

- 1/2 cup chopped nuts (walnuts, almonds, or your choice)

Instructions:

1. Preheat the oven to 350°F (175°C) and line a muffin tin with paper liners.

2. In a bowl, whisk together mashed bananas, melted coconut oil, honey or maple syrup, eggs, and vanilla extract.

3. In another bowl, combine oats, baking powder, cinnamon, and salt.

4. Mix the wet and dry ingredients until well combined. Fold in chopped nuts.

5. Divide the batter evenly among the muffin cups.

6. Bake for about 20-25 minutes, or until a toothpick inserted into the center comes out clean.

7. Allow the muffins to cool before enjoying.

30.Spaghetti Squash with Tomato Basil Sauce

Ingredients:

- 1 medium spaghetti squash
- 2 cups tomato sauce (homemade or store-bought)
- 1/4 cup fresh basil, chopped
- 2 cloves garlic, minced
- 1 tablespoon olive oil
- Salt and pepper to taste
- Grated Parmesan cheese (optional)

Instructions:

1. Preheat the oven to 375°F (190°C).

2. Cut the spaghetti squash in half lengthwise and scoop out the seeds.

3. Place the halves on a baking sheet, cut side up. Drizzle with olive oil and season with salt and pepper.

4. Roast the spaghetti squash in the oven for about 30-40 minutes, until the strands can be easily separated with a fork.

5. While the squash is roasting, heat olive oil in a skillet and sauté minced garlic until fragrant.

6. Add the tomato sauce to the skillet and heat through. Stir in chopped basil.

7. Once the spaghetti squash is cooked, use a fork to scrape the strands out.

8. Serve the spaghetti squash topped with tomato basil sauce. Optionally, sprinkle with grated Parmesan cheese.

31.Creamy Peanut Butter Smoothie

Ingredients:

- 1 cup unsweetened almond milk (or any milk of choice)

- 1 ripe banana

- 2 tablespoons natural peanut butter

- 1 tablespoon chia seeds

- 1/2 teaspoon honey or maple syrup (optional)

- Ice cubes

Instructions:

1. Blend almond milk, ripe banana, peanut butter, chia seeds, honey or maple syrup (if using), and ice cubes until smooth.

2. Pour the smoothie into a glass and enjoy.

32. Roasted Beet and Citrus Salad

Ingredients:

- 2 medium beets, peeled and cubed

- Mixed salad greens (such as spinach, arugula, and/or kale)

- Segments from 1 orange or grapefruit

- 1/4 cup crumbled goat cheese (optional)

- Chopped walnuts or pecans for garnish

For Citrus Vinaigrette:

- Juice of 1 lemon

- Juice of 1 orange or grapefruit

- 2 tablespoons olive oil

- 1 teaspoon honey

- Salt and pepper to taste

Instructions:

1. Preheat the oven to 400°F (200°C).

2. Toss cubed beets with a drizzle of olive oil and roast in the oven until tender and slightly caramelized.

3. Prepare the citrus segments and set aside.

4. In a bowl, whisk together lemon juice, orange or grapefruit juice, olive oil, honey, salt, and pepper to make the vinaigrette.

5. Assemble the salad with mixed greens, roasted beets, citrus segments, crumbled goat cheese (if using), and chopped nuts.

6. Drizzle the citrus vinaigrette over the salad before serving.

33.Herbed Chicken and Vegetable Soup

Ingredients:

- 2 boneless, skinless chicken breasts
- Assorted vegetables (carrots, celery, onions, zucchini), chopped
- 4 cups low-sodium chicken or vegetable broth
- 1 tablespoon olive oil
- 2 cloves garlic, minced
- Fresh herbs (such as thyme, rosemary, parsley)
- Salt and pepper to taste

Instructions:

1. In a pot, heat olive oil over medium heat. Sauté minced garlic until fragrant.
2. Add chopped vegetables and cook until slightly softened.
3. Pour in chicken or vegetable broth and add fresh herbs.
4. Add the chicken breasts and bring the mixture to a simmer. Cook until the chicken is cooked through.
5. Remove the chicken breasts from the pot, shred the meat, and return it to the pot.
6. Season with salt and pepper to taste.

7. Serve the herbed chicken and vegetable soup hot.

34. Walnut-Crusted Salmon with Roasted Vegetables

Ingredients:

- 2 salmon fillets
- 1/2 cup chopped walnuts
- 2 tablespoons Dijon mustard
- 1 tablespoon honey or maple syrup
- 1 teaspoon lemon zest
- Assorted vegetables (such as Brussels sprouts, carrots, red onion)
- Olive oil
- Salt and pepper to taste

Instructions:

1. Preheat the oven to 375°F (190°C).

2. In a bowl, mix chopped walnuts, Dijon mustard, honey or maple syrup, and lemon zest.

3. Season salmon fillets with salt and pepper. Spread the walnut mixture evenly over the top of each fillet.

4. Place the salmon fillets on a baking sheet lined with parchment paper.

5. Toss assorted vegetables with olive oil, salt, and pepper. Spread them on the same baking sheet.

6. Roast in the oven for about 15-20 minutes, or until the salmon is cooked and flakes easily.

7. Serve the walnut-crusted salmon with roasted vegetables.

35.Creamy Cauliflower and Leek Soup

Ingredients:

- 1 head cauliflower, chopped
- 2 leeks, cleaned and chopped
- 1 potato, peeled and diced
- 4 cups vegetable broth
- 1/2 cup unsweetened almond milk (or any milk of choice)
- 2 tablespoons olive oil
- Fresh thyme leaves for garnish
- Salt and pepper to taste

Instructions:

1. In a pot, heat olive oil over medium heat. Sauté chopped leeks until softened.

2. Add chopped cauliflower and diced potato. Cook for a few minutes.

3. Pour in vegetable broth and bring to a boil. Reduce heat and simmer until vegetables are tender.

4. Use an immersion blender to puree the soup until smooth.

5. Stir in almond milk and heat gently. Season with salt and pepper.

6. Serve the creamy cauliflower and leek soup hot, garnished with fresh thyme leaves.

36. Quinoa-Stuffed Portobello Mushrooms

Ingredients:

- 4 large portobello mushrooms, stems removed

- 1 cup cooked quinoa

- 1 cup baby spinach, chopped

- 1/2 cup crumbled feta cheese

- 1/4 cup chopped sun-dried tomatoes

- 2 cloves garlic, minced

- Olive oil

- Salt and pepper to taste

Instructions:

1. Preheat the oven to 375°F (190°C).

2. Brush the portobello mushroom caps with olive oil and season with salt and pepper.

3. In a bowl, combine cooked quinoa, chopped baby spinach, crumbled feta cheese, chopped sun-dried tomatoes, and minced garlic.

4. Stuff each portobello mushroom cap with the quinoa mixture.

5. Place the stuffed mushrooms on a baking sheet and bake for about 20-25 minutes, until the mushrooms are tender.

6. Serve the quinoa-stuffed portobello mushrooms as a main dish or side.

37.Chocolate Avocado Pudding

Ingredients:

- 2 ripe avocados, peeled and pitted

- 1/4 cup unsweetened cocoa powder

- 1/4 cup honey or maple syrup

- 1 teaspoon vanilla extract

- Pinch of salt

- Optional toppings: chopped nuts, berries, shredded coconut

Instructions:

1. In a food processor or blender, combine ripe avocados, cocoa powder, honey or maple syrup, vanilla extract, and a pinch of salt.

2. Blend until smooth and creamy.

3. Taste and adjust sweetness if needed.

4. Divide the chocolate avocado pudding into serving dishes.

5. Top with chopped nuts, berries, or shredded coconut if desired.

38. Asian-Inspired Tofu Stir-Fry

Ingredients:

- 1 block firm tofu, cubed

- Assorted stir-fry vegetables (bell peppers, broccoli, carrots, snap peas)

- 2 tablespoons low-sodium soy sauce or tamari

- 1 tablespoon hoisin sauce

- 1 teaspoon sesame oil

- 1 teaspoon grated fresh ginger

- 2 cloves garlic, minced

- Optional: chopped peanuts or cashews for garnish

Instructions:

1. Press the tofu to remove excess moisture, then cut it into cubes.

2. In a wok or large skillet, heat sesame oil over medium-high heat.

3. Add grated ginger and minced garlic, and sauté briefly until fragrant.

4. Add the tofu cubes and stir-fry until they're lightly browned.

5. Add the stir-fry vegetables and cook until they begin to soften.

6. Drizzle soy sauce or tamari and hoisin sauce over the mixture and toss to combine.

7. Serve the tofu stir-fry with optional chopped nuts on top.

39. Blueberry Almond Chia Pudding

Ingredients:

- 1/4 cup chia seeds

- 1 cup almond milk (or any milk of choice)

- 1/2 teaspoon vanilla extract

- 1 tablespoon honey or maple syrup

- 1/2 cup fresh blueberries

- Sliced almonds for garnish

Instructions:

1. In a jar or bowl, whisk together chia seeds, almond milk, vanilla extract, and honey or maple syrup.

2. Cover and refrigerate for at least 4 hours or overnight, allowing the mixture to thicken.

3. Before serving, give the chia pudding a good stir to break up any clumps.

4. Layer the chia pudding with fresh blueberries in serving glasses.

5. Top with sliced almonds before enjoying.

40.Lemon Garlic Roasted Chicken with Quinoa

Ingredients:

- 2 boneless, skinless chicken breasts

- Zest and juice of 1 lemon

- 2 cloves garlic, minced

- 1 tablespoon olive oil

- Salt and pepper to taste

- 1 cup quinoa, cooked

- Fresh parsley for garnish

Instructions:

1. In a bowl, whisk together lemon zest, lemon juice, minced garlic, olive oil, salt, and pepper.

2. Place the chicken breasts in a resealable plastic bag and pour the marinade over them. Seal the bag and refrigerate for at least 30 minutes.

3. Preheat a grill or grill pan over medium-high heat. Grill the chicken for about 6-7 minutes per side, or until cooked through.

4. Let the chicken rest for a few minutes before slicing.

5. Serve the sliced lemon garlic roasted chicken over cooked quinoa and garnish with fresh parsley.

41.Mediterranean Quinoa Salad

Ingredients:

-   1 cup quinoa, cooked

-   Cherry tomatoes, halved

-   Cucumber, diced

-   Red onion, thinly sliced

-   Kalamata olives, pitted and sliced

-   Feta cheese, crumbled

-   Fresh parsley, chopped

-   Lemon vinaigrette: lemon juice, olive oil, dried oregano, salt, and pepper

Instructions:

1. In a bowl, combine cooked quinoa, halved cherry tomatoes, diced cucumber, thinly sliced red onion,

sliced Kalamata olives, crumbled feta cheese, and chopped fresh parsley.

2. Whisk together lemon juice, olive oil, dried oregano, salt, and pepper to make the vinaigrette.

3. Drizzle the vinaigrette over the salad and toss gently to combine.

4. Serve the Mediterranean quinoa salad as a refreshing side dish or light meal.

42. Stuffed Acorn Squash with Wild Rice and Cranberries

Ingredients:

- 2 acorn squashes, halved and seeds removed
- 1 cup cooked wild rice
- 1/2 cup dried cranberries
- 1/4 cup chopped pecans or walnuts
- 1 tablespoon olive oil
- 1 teaspoon ground cinnamon
- Salt and pepper to taste
- Fresh parsley for garnish

Instructions:

1. Preheat the oven to 375°F (190°C).

2. Rub the inside of each acorn squash half with olive oil and sprinkle with ground cinnamon, salt, and pepper.

3. In a bowl, mix cooked wild rice, dried cranberries, and chopped nuts.

4. Stuff each acorn squash half with the wild rice mixture.

5. Place the stuffed squash halves on a baking sheet and cover with aluminum foil.

6. Bake for about 30-40 minutes, or until the squash is tender.

7. Garnish with fresh parsley before serving.

43. Coconut Mango Chia Seed Parfait

Ingredients:

- 1/4 cup chia seeds

- 1 cup coconut milk (canned or carton)

- 1 tablespoon honey or maple syrup

- 1 ripe mango, diced

- Toasted coconut flakes for garnish

Instructions:

1. In a bowl, whisk together chia seeds, coconut milk, and honey or maple syrup.

2. Cover and refrigerate for at least 4 hours or overnight, allowing the mixture to thicken.

3. Before serving, give the chia pudding a good stir.

4. Layer the chia pudding with diced mango in serving glasses.

5. Top with toasted coconut flakes before enjoying.

44.Roasted Turkey and Cranberry Lettuce Wraps

Ingredients:

- Sliced roasted turkey breast (leftovers or store-bought)

- Lettuce leaves (such as butter lettuce or romaine)

- Cranberry sauce

- Sliced almonds

- Fresh mint leaves

Instructions:

1. Lay out the lettuce leaves on a clean surface.

2. Place slices of roasted turkey on each lettuce leaf.

3. Add a spoonful of cranberry sauce onto the turkey.

4. Sprinkle sliced almonds over the turkey and cranberry.

5. Garnish with fresh mint leaves.

6. Roll up the lettuce leaves to create wraps.

45.Creamy Carrot and Ginger Soup

Ingredients:

- 4 cups chopped carrots

- 1 onion, chopped

- 2 cloves garlic, minced

- 1-inch piece of fresh ginger, peeled and minced

- 4 cups vegetable broth

- 1/2 cup unsweetened almond milk (or any milk of choice)

- 2 tablespoons olive oil

- Fresh cilantro for garnish

- Salt and pepper to taste

Instructions:

1. In a pot, heat olive oil over medium heat. Sauté chopped onion until translucent.

2. Add minced garlic and ginger, and sauté for another minute.

3. Add chopped carrots and vegetable broth. Bring to a boil, then reduce heat and simmer until carrots are tender.

4. Use an immersion blender to puree the soup until smooth.

5. Stir in almond milk and heat gently. Season with salt and pepper.

6. Serve the creamy carrot and ginger soup hot, garnished with fresh cilantro.

46.Quinoa-Stuffed Bell Peppers with Turkey

Ingredients:

- 4 large bell peppers, tops removed and seeds removed

- 1 cup cooked quinoa

- Ground turkey, cooked and seasoned

- 1 cup diced tomatoes (canned or fresh)

- 1/2 cup diced zucchini

- 1/4 cup chopped fresh parsley

- 1 teaspoon dried oregano

- Salt and pepper to taste

- Grated cheese (cheddar or dairy-free alternative), for topping

Instructions:

1. Preheat the oven to 375°F (190°C).

2. In a bowl, combine cooked quinoa, seasoned ground turkey, diced tomatoes, diced zucchini, chopped parsley, dried oregano, salt, and pepper.

3. Stuff each bell pepper with the quinoa and turkey mixture.

4. Place the stuffed peppers in a baking dish. Top with grated cheese.

5. Cover with aluminum foil and bake for about 25-30 minutes. Remove the foil and bake for an additional 10 minutes, until the cheese is melted and bubbly.

6. Allow the stuffed peppers to cool slightly before serving.

47. Raspberry Spinach Salad with Almonds

Ingredients:

- Fresh spinach leaves

- Fresh raspberries

- Sliced almonds, toasted

- Red onion, thinly sliced

- Feta cheese, crumbled

- Balsamic vinaigrette: balsamic vinegar, olive oil, Dijon mustard, honey, salt, and pepper

Instructions:

1. In a bowl, toss together fresh spinach leaves, fresh raspberries, toasted sliced almonds, thinly sliced red onion, and crumbled feta cheese.

2. Whisk together balsamic vinegar, olive oil, Dijon mustard, honey, salt, and pepper to make the vinaigrette.

3. Drizzle the vinaigrette over the salad and gently toss to combine.

4. Serve the raspberry spinach salad as a refreshing and colorful side dish.

48.Baked Sweet Potato Fries

Ingredients:

- Sweet potatoes, peeled and cut into fries

- Olive oil

- Smoked paprika

- Garlic powder

- Salt and pepper to taste

Instructions:

1. Preheat the oven to 425°F (220°C) and line a baking sheet with parchment paper.

2. In a bowl, toss the sweet potato fries with olive oil, smoked paprika, garlic powder, salt, and pepper.

3. Spread the fries in a single layer on the baking sheet.

4. Bake for about 20-25 minutes, turning the fries halfway through, until they're golden and crispy.

5. Serve the baked sweet potato fries as a tasty and nutritious side dish.

49.Chia Seed Energy Bites

Ingredients:

- 1 cup old-fashioned oats
- 1/2 cup almond butter or nut/seed butter of choice
- 1/3 cup honey or maple syrup
- 1/4 cup chia seeds
- 1/4 cup mini chocolate chips or dried fruit
- 1 teaspoon vanilla extract
- Pinch of salt

Instructions:

1. In a bowl, mix together oats, almond butter, honey or maple syrup, chia seeds, chocolate chips or dried fruit, vanilla extract, and a pinch of salt.

2. Refrigerate the mixture for about 30 minutes to make it easier to handle.

3. Roll the mixture into small bites.

4. Place the energy bites on a parchment-lined tray and refrigerate until firm.

5. Store the chia seed energy bites in an airtight container in the refrigerator.

50.Grilled Vegetable and Quinoa Salad

Ingredients:

- 1 cup quinoa, cooked

- Assorted grilled vegetables (zucchini, bell peppers, eggplant, red onion)

- Fresh baby spinach or mixed salad greens

- Balsamic vinaigrette: balsamic vinegar, olive oil, Dijon mustard, honey, salt, and pepper

- Crumbled goat cheese or feta cheese (optional)

Instructions:

1. In a bowl, combine cooked quinoa, grilled vegetables, and fresh baby spinach or mixed salad greens.

2. Whisk together balsamic vinegar, olive oil, Dijon mustard, honey, salt, and pepper to make the vinaigrette.

3. Drizzle the vinaigrette over the salad and toss gently to combine.

4. Top with crumbled goat cheese or feta cheese if desired.

5. Serve the grilled vegetable and quinoa salad as a hearty and satisfying meal.

51.Almond-Crusted Chicken Tenders

Ingredients:

- Boneless, skinless chicken tenders

- Almond meal or ground almonds

- Egg wash (beaten egg with a splash of milk)

- Garlic powder

- Paprika

- Salt and pepper to taste

- Olive oil or cooking spray

Instructions:

1. Preheat the oven to 400°F (200°C) and line a baking sheet with parchment paper.

2. In a shallow bowl, mix almond meal with garlic powder, paprika, salt, and pepper.

3. Dip each chicken tender into the egg wash and then coat with the almond mixture.

4. Place the coated chicken tenders on the baking sheet.

5. Drizzle or spray olive oil over the chicken tenders.

6. Bake for about 15-20 minutes, or until the chicken is cooked through and the coating is crispy.

7. Serve the almond-crusted chicken tenders with a side of dipping sauce.

52. Mediterranean Chickpea Buddha Bowl

Ingredients:

- Cooked quinoa or brown rice

- Chickpeas, cooked and seasoned

- Sliced cucumber

- Cherry tomatoes, halved

- Kalamata olives, pitted and sliced

- Red onion, thinly sliced

- Hummus for drizzling

- Lemon-tahini dressing: tahini, lemon juice, water, garlic, salt, and pepper

Instructions:

1. In a bowl or plate, arrange cooked quinoa or brown rice as the base.

2. Top with seasoned chickpeas, sliced cucumber, halved cherry tomatoes, sliced Kalamata olives, and thinly sliced red onion.

3. Drizzle hummus over the bowl.

4. Whisk together tahini, lemon juice, water, minced garlic, salt, and pepper to make the lemon-tahini dressing.

5. Drizzle the dressing over the Buddha bowl before enjoying.

53. Roasted Vegetable and Hummus Wrap

Ingredients:

- Whole grain or gluten-free wraps

- Roasted vegetables (bell peppers, zucchini, eggplant, red onion)

- Hummus

- Baby spinach or mixed salad greens

- Sliced avocado

- Sunflower seeds or pumpkin seeds for crunch

Instructions:

1. Lay out the wraps on a clean surface.

2. Spread a generous layer of hummus over each wrap.

3. Layer with roasted vegetables, baby spinach or mixed salad greens, sliced avocado, and sunflower or pumpkin seeds.

4. Roll up the wraps tightly, tucking in the sides as you go.

5. Slice the wraps in half and serve as a satisfying and nutritious meal.

54. Mediterranean Quinoa-Stuffed Eggplant

Ingredients:

- 2 large eggplants

- 1 cup cooked quinoa

- Chopped cherry tomatoes

- Chopped cucumber

- Chopped red onion

- Chopped fresh parsley

- Crumbled feta cheese (optional)

- Lemon-tahini dressing: tahini, lemon juice, olive oil, garlic, salt, and pepper

Instructions:

1. Preheat the oven to 375°F (190°C).

2. Cut the eggplants in half lengthwise and scoop out the flesh to create a hollow shell.

3. Rub the eggplant shells with olive oil and sprinkle with salt and pepper. Place them on a baking sheet.

4. In a bowl, mix cooked quinoa, chopped cherry tomatoes, chopped cucumber, chopped red onion, chopped parsley, and crumbled feta cheese (if using).

5. Fill each eggplant shell with the quinoa mixture.

6. Bake in the oven for about 25-30 minutes, until the eggplant is tender and the filling is heated through.

7. Drizzle with lemon-tahini dressing before serving.

55. Creamy Broccoli and Potato Soup

Ingredients:

- 2 cups chopped broccoli florets
- 2 large potatoes, peeled and diced
- 1 onion, chopped
- 2 cloves garlic, minced
- 4 cups vegetable broth
- 1/2 cup unsweetened almond milk (or any milk of choice)
- 1 tablespoon olive oil
- Fresh chives for garnish
- Salt and pepper to taste

Instructions:

1. In a pot, heat olive oil over medium heat. Sauté chopped onion until translucent.

2. Add minced garlic and sauté for another minute.

3. Add diced potatoes and vegetable broth. Bring to a boil, then reduce heat and simmer until potatoes are tender.

4. Add chopped broccoli and continue simmering until broccoli is cooked.

5. Use an immersion blender to puree the soup until smooth.

6. Stir in almond milk and heat gently. Season with salt and pepper.

7. Serve the creamy broccoli and potato soup hot, garnished with fresh chives.

56. Tropical Quinoa Salad with Mango and Avocado

Ingredients:

- 1 cup cooked quinoa

- Ripe mango, diced

- Ripe avocado, diced

- Sliced red bell pepper

- Sliced red onion

- Chopped fresh cilantro

- Lime vinaigrette: lime juice, olive oil, honey, cumin, salt, and pepper

Instructions:

1. In a bowl, combine cooked quinoa, diced mango, diced avocado, sliced red bell pepper, sliced red onion, and chopped cilantro.

2. Whisk together lime juice, olive oil, honey, cumin, salt, and pepper to make the vinaigrette.

3. Drizzle the vinaigrette over the salad and gently toss to combine.

4. Serve the tropical quinoa salad as a refreshing and colorful side dish.

57.Apple Cinnamon Overnight Oats

Ingredients:

- 1/2 cup rolled oats

- 1/2 cup unsweetened almond milk (or any milk of choice)

- 1/2 cup unsweetened applesauce

- 1 teaspoon honey or maple syrup

- 1/2 teaspoon ground cinnamon

- Chopped apples for topping

- Chopped walnuts for topping

Instructions:

1. In a jar or container, combine rolled oats, almond milk, applesauce, honey or maple syrup, and ground cinnamon.

2. Stir well to combine all ingredients.

3. Cover and refrigerate the mixture overnight.

4. In the morning, give the overnight oats a good stir.

5. Top with chopped apples and chopped walnuts before enjoying.

58.Spinach and Mushroom Omelette

Ingredients:

- 3 large eggs

- Handful of baby spinach

- Sliced mushrooms

- Chopped onion

- Grated low-fat cheese (cheddar or Swiss)

- Salt and pepper to taste

- Olive oil

Instructions:

1. In a bowl, whisk the eggs and season with salt and pepper.

2. In a non-stick skillet, heat olive oil over medium heat.

3. Sauté the chopped onion and sliced mushrooms until they soften.

4. Add the baby spinach and cook until wilted.

5. Pour the whisked eggs into the skillet, tilting to spread them evenly.

6. Allow the omelette to cook until set, then sprinkle the grated cheese over one half.

7. Carefully fold the other half of the omelette over the cheese side.

8. Cook for another minute until the cheese is melted.

9. Slide the omelette onto a plate and serve.

59. Lentil and Vegetable Curry

Ingredients:

- 1 cup cooked lentils (green or red)

- Assorted vegetables (carrots, bell peppers, peas, etc.)

- 1 onion, chopped

- 2 cloves garlic, minced

- 1 tablespoon curry powder
- 1 teaspoon ground cumin
- 1 teaspoon ground coriander
- 1/2 teaspoon turmeric
- 1 can (14 oz) coconut milk
- Olive oil
- Salt and pepper to taste
- Fresh cilantro for garnish

Instructions:

1. In a pot, heat olive oil over medium heat. Sauté chopped onion until translucent.

2. Add minced garlic and sauté until fragrant.

3. Add curry powder, ground cumin, ground coriander, and turmeric. Stir to coat the onion and garlic.

4. Add assorted vegetables and cooked lentils. Stir to combine.

5. Pour in the coconut milk and simmer until the vegetables are tender.

6. Season with salt and pepper.

7. Serve the lentil and vegetable curry over rice or quinoa, and garnish with fresh cilantro.

60.Cinnamon Raisin Oatmeal

Ingredients:

- 1/2 cup old-fashioned oats

- 1 cup water or milk (dairy or non-dairy)

- Pinch of salt

- 1/2 teaspoon ground cinnamon

- Handful of raisins

- Chopped nuts (walnuts, almonds) for topping

- Honey or maple syrup for drizzling

Instructions:

1. In a pot, bring water or milk to a boil.

2. Stir in the oats, salt, and ground cinnamon.

3. Reduce the heat to low and simmer, stirring occasionally, until the oats are cooked and the mixture thickens.

4. Stir in the raisins and cook for an additional minute.

5. Remove from heat and let the oatmeal sit for a minute.

6. Serve the oatmeal in bowls, topped with chopped nuts and a drizzle of honey or maple syrup.

61.Greek Yogurt Parfait with Berries and Granola

Ingredients:

- Plain Greek yogurt

- Assorted berries (strawberries, blueberries, raspberries)

- Granola (store-bought or homemade)

- Honey for drizzling

Instructions:

1. In glasses or bowls, layer plain Greek yogurt, assorted berries, and granola.

2. Drizzle honey over each layer for added sweetness.

3. Repeat the layers until the glasses are filled.

4. Serve the Greek yogurt parfait as a delicious and satisfying breakfast or snack.

62.Roasted Butternut Squash Soup

Ingredients:

- 1 small butternut squash, peeled, seeded, and cubed

- 1 onion, chopped

- 2 cloves garlic, minced

- 4 cups vegetable broth

- 1/2 cup unsweetened almond milk (or any milk of choice)

- 1 teaspoon ground cinnamon

- Pinch of nutmeg

- Olive oil

- Salt and pepper to taste

- Pumpkin seeds for garnish

Instructions:

1. Preheat the oven to 400°F (200°C).

2. Toss cubed butternut squash with olive oil, salt, and pepper. Spread on a baking sheet and roast for about 25-30 minutes, until tender and slightly caramelized.

3. In a pot, heat olive oil over medium heat. Sauté chopped onion until translucent.

4. Add minced garlic and sauté until fragrant.

5. Add the roasted butternut squash, vegetable broth, ground cinnamon, and nutmeg. Bring to a simmer and cook for a few minutes.

6. Use an immersion blender to puree the soup until smooth.

7. Stir in almond milk and heat gently. Season with salt and pepper.

8. Serve the roasted butternut squash soup hot, garnished with pumpkin seeds.

63. Tuna and White Bean Salad

Ingredients:

- Canned tuna, drained and flaked

- Canned white beans, drained and rinsed

- Chopped cucumber

- Chopped red onion

- Chopped fresh parsley

- Lemon juice

- Olive oil

- Dijon mustard

- Salt and pepper to taste

Instructions:

1. In a bowl, combine flaked tuna, white beans, chopped cucumber, chopped red onion, and chopped parsley.

2. In a separate small bowl, whisk together lemon juice, olive oil, Dijon mustard, salt, and pepper to make the dressing.

3. Pour the dressing over the salad and toss gently to combine.

4. Serve the tuna and white bean salad as a protein-packed and satisfying meal.

64. Veggie and Hummus Wrap

Ingredients:

- Whole grain or gluten-free wraps

- Hummus

- Sliced avocado

- Sliced bell peppers

- Sliced cucumber

- Shredded carrots

- Baby spinach or mixed salad greens

Instructions:

1. Lay out the wraps on a clean surface.

2. Spread a generous layer of hummus over each wrap.

3. Layer with sliced avocado, sliced bell peppers, sliced cucumber, shredded carrots, and baby spinach or mixed salad greens.

4. Roll up the wraps tightly and slice in half.

5. Serve the veggie and hummus wraps as a quick and nutritious meal.

65. Mixed Berry Smoothie Bowl

Ingredients:

- Assorted frozen berries (strawberries, blueberries, raspberries)

- Banana, sliced

- Unsweetened almond milk (or any milk of choice)

- Greek yogurt

- Toppings: sliced bananas, granola, chia seeds, shredded coconut

Instructions:

1. In a blender, blend frozen berries, sliced banana, almond milk, and a dollop of Greek yogurt until smooth.

2. Pour the smoothie into a bowl.

3. Top with sliced bananas, granola, chia seeds, and shredded coconut for added texture and flavor.

4. Enjoy the mixed berry smoothie bowl as a satisfying breakfast or snack.

66.Quinoa-Stuffed Bell Peppers with Black Beans

Ingredients:

- 4 large bell peppers, tops removed and seeds removed

- 1 cup cooked quinoa

- 1 can black beans, drained and rinsed

- Corn kernels (fresh, frozen, or canned)

- Diced tomatoes

- Chopped fresh cilantro

- Ground cumin

- Salt and pepper to taste

- Shredded cheddar cheese (optional)

Instructions:

1. Preheat the oven to 375°F (190°C).

2. Place the bell peppers on a baking dish.

3. In a bowl, combine cooked quinoa, black beans, corn kernels, diced tomatoes, chopped cilantro, ground cumin, salt, and pepper.

4. Fill each bell pepper with the quinoa and black bean mixture.

5. If using, top with shredded cheddar cheese.

6. Cover the baking dish with aluminum foil and bake for about 25-30 minutes.

7. Remove the foil and bake for an additional 10 minutes, until the peppers are tender and the cheese is melted (if using).

8. Allow the stuffed peppers to cool slightly before serving.

67.Greek Lentil Salad

Ingredients:

- 1 cup cooked green lentils

- Chopped cucumber

- Chopped red bell pepper

- Chopped red onion

- Kalamata olives, pitted and sliced

- Feta cheese, crumbled

- Chopped fresh parsley

- Greek vinaigrette: red wine vinegar, olive oil, dried oregano, garlic, salt, and pepper

Instructions:

1. In a bowl, combine cooked green lentils, chopped cucumber, chopped red bell pepper, chopped red onion, sliced Kalamata olives, crumbled feta cheese, and chopped fresh parsley.

2. Whisk together red wine vinegar, olive oil, dried oregano, minced garlic, salt, and pepper to make the Greek vinaigrette.

3. Drizzle the vinaigrette over the salad and toss gently to combine.

4. Serve the Greek lentil salad as a protein-rich and flavorful dish.

68. Baked Apple Oatmeal Cups

Ingredients:

- 2 cups old-fashioned oats

- 1 teaspoon ground cinnamon

- 1/2 teaspoon ground nutmeg

- Pinch of salt

- 2 cups unsweetened applesauce

- 1/4 cup honey or maple syrup

- 1/2 cup chopped nuts (walnuts, almonds)

- Raisins or dried cranberries

Instructions:

1. Preheat the oven to 350°F (175°C) and grease a muffin tin.

2. In a bowl, mix oats, ground cinnamon, ground nutmeg, and a pinch of salt.

3. Add unsweetened applesauce, honey or maple syrup, chopped nuts, and raisins or dried cranberries. Stir to combine.

4. Spoon the mixture into the muffin tin, filling each cup to the top.

5. Bake for about 20-25 minutes, until the oatmeal cups are set and golden on top.

6. Allow the oatmeal cups to cool before removing from the tin.

69.Berry and Almond Breakfast Parfait

Ingredients:

- Greek yogurt

- Assorted berries (strawberries, blueberries, raspberries)

- Almond butter or chopped almonds

- Honey or maple syrup

- Granola

Instructions:

1. In glasses or bowls, layer Greek yogurt, assorted berries, and almond butter or chopped almonds.

2. Drizzle honey or maple syrup over each layer for sweetness.

3. Repeat the layers until the glasses are filled.

4. Top with granola for added crunch and texture.

5. Serve the berry and almond breakfast parfait as a delicious and wholesome breakfast.

70.Lemon Herb Grilled Salmon

Ingredients:

- Salmon fillets

- Lemon zest and juice

- Fresh herbs (such as dill, parsley, or thyme), chopped

- Olive oil

- Salt and pepper to taste

Instructions:

1. In a bowl, mix together lemon zest, lemon juice, chopped fresh herbs, olive oil, salt, and pepper.

2. Place the salmon fillets in a resealable plastic bag and pour the marinade over them. Seal the bag and refrigerate for at least 30 minutes.

3. Preheat a grill or grill pan over medium-high heat. Grill the salmon for about 4-5 minutes per side, or until cooked through.

4. Serve the lemon herb grilled salmon with a side of steamed vegetables or a salad.

71. Quinoa and Black Bean Stuffed Portobello Mushrooms

Ingredients:

- Portobello mushrooms, stems removed

- 1 cup cooked quinoa

- 1 can black beans, drained and rinsed

- Chopped bell peppers

- Chopped red onion

- Chopped fresh cilantro

- Ground cumin

- Olive oil

- Salt and pepper to taste

- Grated cheese (cheddar or dairy-free alternative), for topping

Instructions:

1. Preheat the oven to 375°F (190°C).

2. Place the portobello mushrooms on a baking sheet.

3. In a bowl, combine cooked quinoa, black beans, chopped bell peppers, chopped red onion, chopped cilantro, ground cumin, olive oil, salt, and pepper.

4. Fill each portobello mushroom cap with the quinoa and black bean mixture.

5. Top with grated cheese.

6. Bake in the oven for about 20-25 minutes, until the mushrooms are tender and the cheese is melted.

7. Allow the stuffed mushrooms to cool slightly before serving.

72.Creamy Avocado Pasta

Ingredients:

- Whole grain or gluten-free pasta

- Ripe avocados, peeled and pitted

- Fresh basil leaves

- Lemon juice

- Garlic, minced

- Olive oil

- Salt and pepper to taste

- Cherry tomatoes, halved

Instructions:

1. Cook the pasta according to package instructions. Drain and set aside.

2. In a food processor, blend ripe avocados, fresh basil leaves, lemon juice, minced garlic, olive oil, salt, and pepper until smooth and creamy.

3. Toss the cooked pasta with the creamy avocado sauce.

4. Gently fold in halved cherry tomatoes.

5. Serve the creamy avocado pasta as a flavorful and nourishing meal.

73. Mixed Bean and Corn Salad

Ingredients:

- Assorted canned beans (black beans, kidney beans, cannellini beans), drained and rinsed

- Corn kernels (fresh, frozen, or canned)

- Chopped bell peppers (assorted colors)

- Chopped red onion

- Chopped fresh cilantro

- Lime juice

- Olive oil

- Ground cumin

- Salt and pepper to taste

Instructions:

1. In a bowl, combine assorted beans, corn kernels, chopped bell peppers, chopped red onion, and chopped cilantro.

2. Whisk together lime juice, olive oil, ground cumin, salt, and pepper to make the dressing.

3. Drizzle the dressing over the bean and corn salad and toss gently to combine.

4. Serve the mixed bean and corn salad as a protein-packed side dish or light meal.

74. Sweet Potato and Black Bean Tacos

Ingredients:

- Whole grain or corn tortillas

- Roasted sweet potatoes, diced

- Canned black beans, drained and rinsed

- Sliced avocado

- Sliced red onion

- Chopped fresh cilantro

- Lime wedges

- Greek yogurt or dairy-free yogurt (for topping)

- Ground cumin

- Smoked paprika

- Salt and pepper to taste

Instructions:

1. Warm the tortillas according to package instructions.

2. In a bowl, mix diced roasted sweet potatoes with drained black beans.

3. Season with ground cumin, smoked paprika, salt, and pepper.

4. Fill each tortilla with the sweet potato and black bean mixture.

5. Top with sliced avocado, sliced red onion, chopped cilantro, and a dollop of Greek yogurt or dairy-free yogurt.

6. Serve the sweet potato and black bean tacos with lime wedges for squeezing.

75.Grilled Chicken and Veggie Skewers

Ingredients:

- Chicken breast, cut into cubes

- Assorted vegetables (bell peppers, zucchini, red onion, cherry tomatoes)

- Olive oil

- Fresh lemon juice

- Garlic, minced

- Fresh herbs (such as rosemary, thyme, or oregano), chopped

- Salt and pepper to taste

Instructions:

1. In a bowl, mix olive oil, fresh lemon juice, minced garlic, chopped fresh herbs, salt, and pepper to create a marinade.

2. Thread the chicken cubes and assorted vegetables onto skewers.

3. Brush the skewers with the marinade.

4. Preheat a grill or grill pan over medium-high heat. Grill the skewers for about 10-12 minutes, turning occasionally, until the chicken is cooked through and the vegetables are charred and tender.

5. Serve the grilled chicken and veggie skewers with a side salad or whole grain.

76. Mediterranean Brown Rice Salad

Ingredients:

- Cooked brown rice

- Chopped cucumber

- Chopped red bell pepper

- Kalamata olives, pitted and sliced

- Crumbled feta cheese

- Chopped fresh parsley

- Lemon vinaigrette: lemon juice, olive oil, Dijon mustard, garlic, salt, and pepper

Instructions:

1. In a bowl, combine cooked brown rice, chopped cucumber, chopped red bell pepper, sliced Kalamata olives, crumbled feta cheese, and chopped fresh parsley.

2. Whisk together lemon juice, olive oil, Dijon mustard, minced garlic, salt, and pepper to make the vinaigrette.

3. Drizzle the lemon vinaigrette over the salad and toss gently to combine.

4. Serve the Mediterranean brown rice salad as a refreshing and nutritious dish.

77.Mango and Quinoa Salad

Ingredients:

- Cooked quinoa

- Ripe mango, diced

- Sliced red bell pepper

- Sliced red onion

- Chopped fresh cilantro

- Lime juice

- Olive oil

- Ground cumin

- Salt and pepper to taste

Instructions:

1. In a bowl, combine cooked quinoa, diced ripe mango, sliced red bell pepper, sliced red onion, and chopped fresh cilantro.

2. Whisk together lime juice, olive oil, ground cumin, salt, and pepper to create a dressing.

3. Drizzle the dressing over the salad and toss gently to combine.

4. Serve the mango and quinoa salad as a vibrant and flavorful side dish.

78.Broccoli and Almond Soup

Ingredients:

- 2 cups broccoli florets

- 1 onion, chopped

- 2 cloves garlic, minced

- 4 cups vegetable broth

- 1/2 cup unsweetened almond milk (or any milk of choice)

- 1/4 cup almonds, toasted and chopped

- Olive oil

- Salt and pepper to taste

Instructions:

1. In a pot, heat olive oil over medium heat. Sauté chopped onion until translucent.

2. Add minced garlic and sauté until fragrant.

3. Add broccoli florets and vegetable broth. Bring to a boil, then reduce heat and simmer until broccoli is tender.

4. Use an immersion blender to puree the soup until smooth.

5. Stir in almond milk and heat gently. Season with salt and pepper.

6. Serve the broccoli and almond soup hot, garnished with chopped toasted almonds.

79.Grilled Veggie Wrap with Hummus

Ingredients:

- Whole grain or gluten-free wraps
- Hummus
- Grilled vegetables (zucchini, eggplant, bell peppers)
- Baby spinach or mixed salad greens
- Sliced red onion
- Sliced avocado

Instructions:

1. Lay out the wraps on a clean surface.

2. Spread a layer of hummus over each wrap.

3. Layer with grilled vegetables, baby spinach or mixed salad greens, sliced red onion, and sliced avocado.

4. Roll up the wraps tightly, tucking in the sides as you go.

5. Slice the wraps in half and serve as a satisfying and flavorful meal.

80.Berry Chia Pudding

Ingredients:

*   1/4 cup chia seeds

*   1 cup unsweetened almond milk (or any milk of choice)

*   Mixed berries (strawberries, blueberries, raspberries)

*   Honey or maple syrup (optional)

*   Chopped nuts (almonds, walnuts) for topping

Instructions:

1. In a jar or container, mix chia seeds and almond milk. Stir well.

2. Refrigerate the mixture for a few hours or overnight, until it thickens into a pudding-like consistency.

3. Layer the chia pudding with mixed berries in serving glasses.

4. If desired, drizzle honey or maple syrup over each layer.

5. Top with chopped nuts for added crunch.

6. Enjoy the berry chia pudding as a delightful dessert or breakfast.

= THE END =

We appreciate you selecting this book! We hope your expectations were fulfilled or surpassed.

Please think about posting a review on social media if you liked our book. We value your opinion because it enables us to make improvements to our goods and services for future clients.

We want to thank you once more for your support and send our best to you.